I Hurt Like Hell

We Have All Heard of Fibromyalgia, Now Hear It from Someone Who Lives It Every Day

by

Annette L. Jackson

DORRANCE PUBLISHING CO., INC.
PITTSBURGH, PENNSYLVANIA 15222

Dorrance Publishing Co., Inc.
701 Smithfield Street
Pittsburgh, PA 15222
Visit our website at *www.dorrancebookstore.com*

ISBN: 978-1-4349-1284-8
eISBN: 978-1-4349-7026-8

I Hurt Like Hell

We have all heard of fibromyalgia. Now, hear it from someone who lives it every day.

By Annette L. Jackson

Dedication

To my parents, who are gone, but not forgotten.
To my family for being more than I could ask for.
To my doctor, who always listened and always believed my pain
was real.
To my best friend, who continues to be my best friend and
confidant.
To my husband, without his love and support this could not
have been possible.
Thank you to my ex-husband for making me realize the only
person I can truly count on is me.
To all those who suffer from FMS,
You inspire me and continue to inspire me every day you fight
this disease.

I Hurt Like Hell

How my life was turned upside down with fibromyalgia, one of the most misunderstood and complex conditions in today's society.

Foreword

Fibromyalgia.

You may have heard about it, you may know someone who has it, or you yourself may have this condition. The truth is the more you hear about FMS, the more you find that many people have it. Just thirteen years ago when I was first diagnosed, there was very little information available to me, and there were very few options for treatment. My first prescription was a muscle relaxer and my first treatment was ultrasound therapy to my neck and shoulders. I continue to work and do all the things I enjoyed. It felt like I had a little whiplash and pain in my fingertips.

Fast forward to the year 2010.

The word "fibromyalgia" seems to be everywhere. Everyone knows of someone who has it and there are several new medications for treatment. There are also more options for physical therapy.

Currently, I am unable to work and unable to do most of the things I used to enjoy. Even though I was told this disease was not progressive, I seem to have gotten only worse. I decided to write this book to reach out to those who suffer from fibromyalgia or chronic pain. They may feel that no one around them understands their pain or cares about it. They may feel alone, depressed, and desperate. I just want to say I do feel your pain, I do care, and you're not alone. Your pain is real and your emotions are real. Maybe keep this book close to your heart and when you feel no one understands you, open it up and remember that I do. I live it every day.

Chapter One
Something Feels Different

Fibromyalgia, it seems to begin the same way for all of us–a pain here or a sore muscle there. Maybe you have migraine or pain in your fingers and toes. There could be a bruise for no reason or a sore that doesn't heal. Whatever it is, we feel like something's going on inside of us and we don't know what to do about it. To begin with, we may take Tylenol or Advil, or use one of the many creams and ointments available at the drugstore. None of these products seem to help us feel any better or alleviate the pain.

Then other factors begin to appear. It becomes harder and harder to get to sleep or stay asleep. No position feels comfortable and aches and pains that were with us during the day are also there at night. When you do wake up in the morning, you almost feel like you've been run over by a truck. You still ache, you still feel unrested, and you're wondering how you're going to get through another day. These episodes will go on for a while until finally one day you decide to make an appointment with your doctor.

If you do find yourself talking to friends and family about how you feel, you will get all kinds of advice. Someone will recommend physical therapy, a chiropractor, or other alternative medicines such as acupuncture, massage, or herbal supplements. There may even be ads in a magazine or infomercials on television promising you that they can stop your pain or discomfort. Be careful of some of these alternative medicines because most of these are not covered by insurance and can be quite costly. For instance, a visit to the chiropractor may make the pain better, but at $80 a visit how often could you afford to go? Don't misunderstand me. I think people do benefit from chiropractic care, but for fibromyalgia it does not seem to get to the root of the pain.

I recently have discovered in some large shopping malls and at the airport, there are places that give ten-minute massages. These are usually conducted by Asian people who seem to really know about muscle pain and trigger point release. The ones I have done were $10 for ten minutes and was the best $10 I have spent.

Just seeing these places popping up and seeing so many commercials about pain relief makes me think people are starting to accept this disease as real. I finally feel like we have a voice and we're being heard. Just want to caution you, though: Use these facilities at your own risk. I have been to massage therapists who gave me a full-body massage for one hour and I left hurting so bad. They were too rough, using their elbows instead of their hands to massage. One time, I went to the chiropractor and he crossed both my arms across my chest and kneeled down on my chest and popped my back. I thought I was paralyzed and never did that again.

I like using a hot tub, but as far as giving me relief, I can't really say. I will say that a hot tub or hot shower always feels good, but does not give me long-term pain relief. I actually get a lot of relief from ice packs on my back. I think this is because most of my pain is nerve pain. It just feels like my nerve endings are on fire and ice packs seem to cool them down. I sleep on my stomach and sometimes wrap an ice pack in a towel and lay it across my back and then fall asleep. Be careful not to leave the ice pack on bare skin for longer than directed by a physician. That also goes for other home remedies for pain relief, including pain patches, heat wraps, TENS unit, and ice packs.

Chapter Two
The Fibromyalgia Pain

There are many words I could think of to describe the pain of fibromyalgia. Some of the first ones that come to mind are stabbing, burning, gnawing, unrelenting, pulling, and crawling. When I'm in the throes of pain, I can't think or move. My body's throbbing as if it were wrapped up in pain. Sometimes, I can be found curled up in a fetal position on the floor.

I try so hard to get at my trigger points. I want to push on them, massage them, stick needles in them, anything to get relief. I have even taken a hammer to my back and neck muscles when they are knotted up. Acupuncture did not help. I use various trigger-point-release items sold online or in stores. Most of those items have four or six prongs. I have used pain patches with some relief. I also use a TENS unit almost twenty-four hours a day. I believe it has given me the most relief outside of pain pills.

Sometimes, water from the shower hurts and sometimes it feels good. With the bipolar, I just can't get too overheated. I have a massage chair, and I have two handheld massagers. Sometimes I use them so long that it hurts my arm to hold it anymore. If I get a professional massage, I prefer a ten-minute sitting massage as opposed to the sixty laying-down massage. The sixty-minute massage is usually deep tissue and I end up extremely sore the next day.

I have had this pain almost every day for thirteen years. Usually, my pain level is between six and eight, but I have had many days with a ten plus. On those days when it's been a ten, I have wished for God to just take me. The pain is so unbearable and so unrelenting it doesn't even seem human. I'm not saying I'm suicidal; I just can't take that much pain and live through it. I have even imagined that I have a morphine drip and it has slowly taken the pain away. That's all I can do until I fall asleep. Sleeping is the only way I can survive that much pain. Sometimes, I'm not even sure if I can take this much pain the rest of my life, but I guess I'll have to.

The one breakthrough medication I have for that much pain is methadone. It takes a while to kick in, but it does finally relieve the pain. The only problem though is that it keeps me awake for 24 to 48 hours. So I can't take it that often because I can't put my muscles through that. Plus, methadone carries a lot of stigma with it, so I don't tell anyone I take it. It is a very good analgesic with very few side effects on the body. I have read that methadone is stored in the liver to be used at a later time.

The only other way I help with the pain is just to be asleep. It's hard for me to get to sleep at night, and usually I fall asleep about one or two early in the morning. If I get to sleep by two, I will get up about ten. If it wasn't for Ambien or Lunesta, I would never fall asleep. In order to enjoy my evening, I try to take a nap between five and seven in the evening. I don't always get a nap, but I feel better if I do. I also take something for anxiety. The disease of FMS alone is enough to give anyone anxiety. Between the chronic pain and the bipolar disorder and being alone, that's a lot to deal with every day. Sometimes, I'm just sad and I cry. I find crying to be a good release of tension and anxiety. Laughter is also a good release of tension and anxiety, so I will put in a funny movie or read something funny.

Chapter Three
The Only Time I Don't Feel Pain Is When I'm Asleep

I don't say this to sound dramatic or to say that FMS pain is worse than in any other disease. I just know this is true for me. In the beginning, my pain was bad but did not define me or my lifestyle. I continued to work and enjoy my social life; basically, not much had changed. I can honestly say now, as the years progress, that there is less and less I can do. I find myself telling my husband, "I can't even do what I did six months ago."

I was diagnosed in 1997. I may have mentioned that in another chapter. I experience some pain and fatigue, but nothing compared to what I have now. In 2003, I went on vacation with my sister and her children. We went to Florida and I was involved in a lot of activity. We went to the beach, amusement park and also to a water park. It was a very good trip, the only time I realized I had some fatigue was on the flight home. Also, I don't recall having very much pain. In 2004, I took a trip with my brother and his family, a similar kind of vacation; we went to the amusement park and a water park. I recall having more fatigue with this trip. When I got back home, I had to end up taking two more extra days off to rest. I think I even fell asleep in my clothes I was so exhausted.

By 2005, that was it, my husband and I took a road trip to Illinois and by the time I got home, I was overcome with so much pain and fatigue that I never returned to work. Even though I was not working, I still had severe pain and fatigue. Over the years, I have noticed the FMS is steadily getting worse. No matter what medicine I take or how much exercise I get, there is just no relief from the pain. I try to eat healthy, even tried yoga and Pilates. I have tried acupuncture, deep tissue massage, trigger point injections, and spent lots of money on home remedies. I have a shiatsu chair massager and several handheld massagers. Still I find the only relief is sleep.

I think the hardest thing is that my mind is still sharp. I tried to read and learn something new every day. I sit here and think of things I used to do that I enjoyed so much. For instance, going to the movies, going to the beach, shopping, and so on. It's kind of a weird feeling, your mind thinks you can do all these things, then your body lets you know that you can't. Even when I attempt to do simple household chores, it can seem like I'm attempting to climb Mount Everest. It's hard for anyone to understand this, but some days by the time I get up and get a shower and dressed, it's almost dinner time. The day is gone and it's time to get ready for bed. Getting to sleep is another hard part of my day. Some nights it can take hours, and some nights I don't sleep at all because of pain.

I know my condition could be worse and I have been lucky to have been blessed with a supportive husband, family, and friends. I also have a caring doctor who believes in my pain and a wonderful therapist whom I see every week. I have had to do a great deal of reading on accepting my disease and facing it with courage. I heard someone say a while back, the courage doesn't mean you don't have fear, but you move forward despite the fear.

I don't know how much further my FMS will progress. Even though much information about FMS says it is not a progressive disease, I feel I have progressively gotten worse. So, yes, the only time I don't feel pain is when I'm asleep. I'm just glad I'm alive and able to feel anything. There are other feelings that I feel in addition to the pain: love, joy, laughter, hurt, and sadness. Feelings that are a part of all us. For all the darkness and the loneliness I sometimes feel with FMS, there are bright spots where I experience love and laughter and the spirit of belonging. And for this I am thankful.

Chapter Four
Dealing with Public Opinion

Unfortunately, this can be just as hard to deal with as the fibromyalgia itself. Sometimes, I hate to even say I have FMS, preferring just to say I have chronic pain. Even if I don't hear it directly, people do say things under their breath or you find out later from someone else what they said. It hurts, it really does. Not only are you battling all this pain and lack of sleep, but then to hear all the ridicule. Some of it even comes from people you thought were close to you.

These are just a few of the many things I have heard over the years. I am positive I could list more but you get the general idea. I think of all the diseases and conditions out there in the world, and it seems to me that FMS is the most ridiculed and least believed. I have actually prayed that I wish I had cancer or other terminal condition just so I would be treated with compassion and understanding. I am in no way comparing FMS to cancer. I just wish one time someone would give me a hug and tell me it's going to be okay.

I know that there are times I parked in a handicapped zone and people stare at me with disgust. So now I no longer use them. I have wanted to use the power chair at a grocery store, but I don't dare. I just feel too guilty and people make me feel so ashamed. I have heard some of my relatives think I have a prescription drug problem and there is no way I could possibly need all of these medicines. Do I need to remind them that I have FMS and bipolar disease? Friends and coworkers used to say, "You don't look like you're in pain," or "Your pain cannot be that bad." Here are some more comments I have heard: "All you do is complain about pain"; "so-and-so has it and she doesn't complain"; "so-and-so has had it longer and is much worse off than you are."

As if those statements were not hurtful enough, here are some more: "Maybe you're just lazy and don't want to work"; "you always want to lie down and sleep"; "you never want to go anywhere or do anything"; "why don't you clean the house like you used to?"

Since I suffer from bipolar disease, some people have told me that maybe my depression is causing my aches and pains. After all I take all these pills and they don't seem to be helping. Some have said I have a low tolerance for pain. Most of the time, I don't even tell them about the bipolar condition because that carries a stigma all on its own.

Anyway, for now I know this disease is real, the pain is real, the impact it's had on my life and workplace is real, and the impact it's had on my relationships is real. There is currently some research for FMS, but because it is not life-threatening or fatal it sits on the back burner. Fibromyalgia headlines seem to be making their way on to the Internet, magazines, and even on TV. I currently hand out FMS support bands to family, friends, and sometimes strangers. They are pink and crimson. Pink is for women and crimson is for pain. For whatever reason, this disease seems to afflict more women than men.

I have been told it is not a progressive disease, but I have only become worse since my initial diagnosis. I have no idea how bad it will get or if there will be a medication to give me relief. I feel like I am already on chemotherapy. I have thrown up from taking my medicine, I have gotten chills and night sweats, and I have had some of my hair fall out. Most days I'm in pain, I feel weak and lethargic, I can't seem to do anything or enjoy anything. Ninety-nine percent of my time is spent alone for one reason or another.

Chapter Five
Medication

The subject always gets me upset, not because I have anything against medicines, but it's everyone else that seems to. I get enough crap simply for having FMS. Because there is no definite test for FMS and it does not seem to appear on any type of X-ray, most people don't take it seriously. Plus, I get called all kinds of names and I'm given some pretty lame advice. I'm sure those of you who have FMS have heard these before: you're lazy, it's not that bad, just toughen up, you just don't want to work, it's all in your mind, everybody has aches and pains. I wonder if they would say these things if I had cancer or multiple sclerosis or some other debilitating disease. I doubt it.

Now, let's talk about medication. Most of us are prescribed various medications based on our symptoms and the severity of our symptoms. One reason FMS is hard to detect is because most of us have nerve pain. Nerve pain can be extremely painful. Just ask a diabetic who has had diabetic neuropathy. I personally have a lot of nerve pain in my neck, upper back, and along both sides of my rib cage. Sometimes, the pain has been so overwhelming I find the nearest chair or bed and nearly pass out.

Some of us with FMS take medication that is prescribed for cancer-like pain. From what I've read, it seems most FMS patients—including myself—do fairly well with the following kinds of medication: antidepressants, anticonvulsants, muscle relaxers, some form of sleep medication, and some form of breakthrough pain medication. For me that breakthrough pain medication is methadone. I am only prescribed a few at a time and they usually last three to four months. That's because I don't take them every day and I usually don't take a whole one. I usually only take methadone when all else has failed, after I have tried OTC medication, my prescription medication, massage therapy, heat or ice packs, and complete bed rest and sleep. One reason I can't take methadone too often is because I have a paradoxical effect to narcotics or opiates. Instead of relaxing me or causing me drowsiness, they have the opposite effect and keep me awake for 24 to 48 hours. I don't take most of the medicines because of the stigma people attach to many of them.

In the past, I have tried Vicodin, Percocet, Lortab, and Darvocet to name a few, but they did not reduce my pain. Methadone seems to be the only analgesic that works. I also suffer from bipolar disorder, so I have a separate drug regimen for that. For the most part, my medications keep my symptoms under control, but I still have a constant pain level of five to six. If I didn't take my pain medicine and my bipolar medication, I would have above-ten pain every day and probably never sleep. I did try that once because I was sick of all the name-calling. I put my health and my life at risk just because people were calling me a "drug addict." I stopped everything cold turkey and ended up in the hospital. That will never happen again.

I am always so shocked at what people say to me. No matter how severe my pain is, I am told I am a drug addict. I have had people tell me I take the meds to get "high." If I pass out from pain, people will say I have over-medicated myself. It used to bother me, but now I just don't listen to them. They don't know what it's like. They don't have my pain. Even people close to me question my medication all the time. I know my pain is real and I don't have to prove it to anyone. I'm going to take care of myself and do whatever I need to do to ease some of the pain. No one else is going to do it for me and I'm tired of explaining myself. I just have to be strong and just know that my doctor and I know it's real. I am no different than someone on chemotherapy. Nobody's words can hurt me anymore. I have had FMS for about fourteen years now and even though it's getting worse, I can't let it get me down. I still want to enjoy life and be surrounded by family and friends that love me. I know I have lost some people in my life because of this disease or because they didn't want to understand it. But I've also gained a few along this journey.

I guess what I really want to say is don't let anyone convince you that your pain is not real. Find yourself a caring and compassionate doctor. Look online or in your community for FMS support groups. Reach out to family and friends and find that one person you can talk to or cry to when you need to. We did not ask for this disease and I would not wish it on anyone. What more can I say, these are the cards I've been dealt. This was one of my main goals in writing this book. I wanted everyone suffering from this disease to know they are not alone and that they're not crazy. I wanted them to have this book for themselves, family members, and friends, especially those who are newly diagnosed as I know how scary this can be. As of the last statistics I read, there are least 3 to 4,000,000 people in the United States alone who have FMS, and they are mainly women.

Chapter Six
Loneliness

If there's one thing I can say about fibromyalgia, it would be that loneliness is a huge part of it. It's really no one's fault, it just sort of happens. Your friends and family invite you to functions or outings in the beginning. Sometimes you can go and sometimes you can't. But over time as the fibromyalgia gets worse, you find yourself saying no more than yes. Then the invitations become less, the phone rings less, until you realize that you are all alone.

It's kind of a double-edged sword, people don't want to make you feel bad if you can't go, and you don't want to make them feel bad by always saying no. And it doesn't help that stress and emotions make the fibromyalgia pain worse. Sometimes you are afraid of going public for fear that you will have a painful episode. You don't want to find yourself in a situation that you cannot get out of or away from. Just the thought of being confined can cause your pain levels to rise. For me personally, I cannot handle airline seats. From the moment I sit down till the moment I get out of it, my pain level is ten plus. Riding in a car can be painful, but riding in a truck is not as painful. I guess it's the way the seats are designed.

I think this is why I spend a lot of time alone. I tend to change positions, seats, chairs all day long in my house. To some people it might seem odd, but for me it's all about comfort. It sounds crazy but there are actually some homes I hate going to because they have uncomfortable furniture. Some days I'm sad about being alone and some days I'm glad I'm alone by myself. Because

I get so tired of explaining why I need this or why I don't, or why this is comfortable and why this isn't. It's too hard to explain and it's even harder to understand. I have the disease and I still don't know why some things are the way they are.

I have found ways to beat the loneliness by using my free time to learn new things. I try every day to learn at least one thing new either on the Internet or on TV. Just because my body is disabled doesn't mean my mind is. I have a dog that I get out and walk, which helps me in two ways. First it gets me out of the house and exercising, and second, I almost always run into someone to talk to. I really can't even say that I feel lonely because usually I'm so busy. There are some days I wish my husband was home more often, but he works and he likes to play golf. So I want him to do what makes him happy because I will be okay. In all actuality, my friends and family are just a phone call away. I know if I truly needed anyone of them they would be here in an instant, and I'm okay with that. Every once in a while, I will find myself having a pity party, but I really don't like feeling sorry for myself. There are certainly worse things in the world than having fibromyalgia and bipolar disorder.

Of course, I didn't always feel this way. I've had some pretty rough times in my life. I develop an eating disorder at sixteen and that led to a major depression cycle, which held me down for almost twenty-five years. I've been in a psychiatric ward three times, I have tried to commit suicide, and went through a painful divorce in 2000. I would say around 1997 is when I first noticed the signs of chronic pain. At the time my husband and I thought it was just a neck muscle spasm. As time went on, it just never got better and nothing seemed to bring me any relief. My husband seemed to be understanding in the beginning, massaging my neck and trying to make me comfortable. Somewhere along the way, I guess he felt cheated. He did not want a wife that was sick all the time or could not go places. The more my fibromyalgia worsened, the more distant he became.

By 1999, he had developed a relationship through the Internet. He actually began this relationship right after I had a miscarriage. By the year 2000, it was obvious to both of us that the marriage was never going to work. So we filed for separation and eventually a divorce. I remember feeling so afraid. Where was I going to go and how was I going to do it? I had never felt so alone and scared in my whole life. Everything seemed to be happening so fast and I had so much to do. I moved in with a good friend of mine, so I didn't have to live alone. I was able to apply for medical and dental benefits at my job. I knew I couldn't ask for much help from my family because they just didn't have it.

Chapter Seven
Accept, Accept, Accept

I think more than anything, I have had to diagnose my situation. I can't change those things and I cannot change people, but I can change myself. Most of it involves acceptance and gratitude. I have to realize my situation could be so much worse, so much worse.

One of the reasons I'm writing this book is to reach out to those who may be struggling and may not be as fortunate. I just want them to know I understand and I have been there. I want them to have this book so they know someone out there understands their pain, their frustration, there depression, and their hopelessness. I have definitely been there in some days I still go back. I think it's normal to feel okay for a while and then get so depressed you just want to give up. I can only hope that those reading this book have a good pain doctor, a good friend or therapist, and the family support system. I find all those ingredients to be so important.

I don't know if I will ever be able to work again. Maybe my work outlook will have to change. I would love to go back to school and possibly get a degree in psychology so I can help those dealing with FMS or chronic pain, and those who may be dealing with a co-existing mental condition like depression or bipolar. I just want to listen and let them know it will be okay. I can't fix it, but I can give comfort. I want to continue to learn the latest on FMS or chronic pain including new treatments and medication.

If nothing else, those who buy this book can just keep it close or share it with someone in their support system. It just feels good for someone to say, "I understand and I know how you feel." That's the book I looked for when I was first diagnosed. I saw a lot of books written by doctors and experts on the subject of FMS, that they themselves did not have the disease. I needed a book where the author was saying, "I have FMS and I understand."

I have accepted my disease, but I continue to advocate for things to be easier for my condition. I so appreciate anyone else who advocates for me. Even my niece and nephew who are young are aware of my FMS and advocate for me. Then there is the dreaded acceptance that there will be those who don't understand and don't want to. I have lost relationships over my conditions and diseases. Not that having them is my fault, but there will always be those who will think what they will. I don't blame them. I just try to hold my head up and walk away. For the many who don't want to be a part of my life, there will still be someone who does. After all, I am not just my disease and conditions. I am a kind, loving, caring, and intelligent individual. I'm not perfect, but I always try to do the right thing. I have a lot of insight and I can be a good listener. I try every day to be a good wife, sister, and friend. That is all I can do for now. Of course, there will always be those who never accept me, but isn't this true of almost everyone? I think all of us at one time or another have yearned for acceptance.

Chapter Eight
Double Whammy

As if FMS and chronic pain were not enough, I also suffer from bipolar disorder. Some days I just want to throw my hands up and say, "I surrender." It is a lot of work dealing with both of these disorders.

Either one of them on their own would be enough. Tackling both of them at the same time is a huge challenge and takes a lot of energy and patience. You have to have a precise regimen and take care of your mind and body. This includes taking the medicines for the bipolar or chronic pain and nutritional or vitamin supplements. In order to avoid becoming confused when taking medicines, I suggest you get a weekly pill divider. Not only one that separates the days, but also one that separates the time of day. Remember that some of these medicines can cause drowsiness, and you don't want to be drowsy and be in charge of your medication.

Some of the pain medicine can override the bipolar medication. They can make you nauseated and affect your appetite, so make sure you are eating healthy. Because we can't be sure we are always eating healthy, it's important to take multivitamin and multi-mineral supplements. Get plenty of rest and exercise. Keep your personal hygiene up. You may not feel your best, but try to present your best. Most days, I wake up feeling like I've been run over by a truck, but I get up, shower, and get dressed. All of this does not change the fact that I have FMS and bipolar disorder, but I do generally feel better about myself. It's hard but I always try to find the good or the positive in everyday life.

Be gentle and kind to yourself, after all you did not ask for this to happen. You will have days that you don't want to get out of bed, but that's okay. Don't be so hard on yourself. Just use the rest of this day to relax and sleep and try again tomorrow. Sometimes, I get down and depressed, have a pity party, and feel sorry for myself. When I find myself in the situation, I try to distract myself or look at the news on TV and see people living with much worse conditions than mine. It's a funny feeling though, to be held captive in your own body.

I feel like my only real escape is when I am sleeping. I can be or do anything in my dreams. I also find myself going back to a time before I had either of these conditions. That wonderful time before I had so much pain and depression. I can't remember the last time I lay down and just fell asleep. Now, I have to take a sleeping pill or some kind of pill just to make my eyes close and sleep. My mind is constantly going, constantly thinking, and I like learning new things just so I can memorize them. I wish I had a switch that I could turn my brain off and on.

I'm forty-five now and I wish I could remember who I used to be. What kind of person was I? I can't seem to handle anything anymore, either mentally or physically. Nowadays, too much overload on my brain throws me into a tailspin. This is why I watch a lot of movies and browse through the Internet. My mind is the only thing I can still entertain without overdoing it.

There's an old saying, "start low, go slow." I feel like this one very much applies to me now.

Chapter Nine
Don't Give Up

Some days I want to give up. Not because I want to die, but because I can't live with this much pain. Could you imagine pain taking over your entire body and interfering in every aspect of your life? It ruins your relationships and sometimes you lose your job or are forced to quit. When you first get the diagnosis of FMS, you really think it can't be all that bad. Then as the years go on, it becomes apparent that this monster is bigger than you could have imagined. Pain medicine helps, but not completely and not all the time. Plus, if you take medication all the time for the pain, then you end up missing out on life.

You no longer get to have the life you want. It can become so lonely and depressing. You have to be strong in your faith and have faith in those who are helping you. I would be lying if I said I never thought of suicide. I think that is normal considering the disease and the depression. After all, there are other chronic conditions or terminal illnesses where people have thought of suicide. There are some patients who suffer a mental illness along with the fibromyalgia. Imagine having FMS and bipolar together. Your mind could be constantly bombarded with suicidal ideation. You have to learn to deal with these thoughts because you can't control them. You don't want to have suicidal thoughts, but they just keep coming.

I consider myself very lucky because I have a list of people I can call when this happens to me. Instead of acting on the suicidal thought, I phone a family member, close friend, or my physician until it passes. Suicide can never be an option for any of us because that would be so unfair to hurt those we leave behind. I have been told that suicide is a permanent solution to a temporary problem. A long time ago, I did find myself in that position when I was in a lot of pain and I thought the whole world was not listening to me. I took too much pain medication and had to go to the hospital. My family and friends were devastated and it was right then I vowed to never go down that road again. We must always ask for help and we must get over the feeling that we are a burden. If a close family member or friend has an illness we don't think of them as a burden. People with FMS need to realize that their pain is real and we are not a burden to anyone. Even in this busy world, you have to trust that people love you and care about you. Find someone to talk to who will listen to you. Ask if it is okay to call if you need them. Find a good pain doctor and the therapists that will always return your phone call.

Always remind yourself that you are important. Take all your medications as prescribed. If you're having trouble with the side effects or you feel they are not helping, please contact your doctor. In dealing with chronic pain, especially FMS, the relationship between you and your doctors is absolutely so important. The medical community is learning more and more about FMS every day. So that is why I say, "Don't give up." Don't give up on yourself and don't give up on your life.

Chapter Ten
It's not Fair

It seems like the same game every day. The only problem is I never get to win. I wake up, pain starts and then pain lasts the rest of the day. Sometimes, I even lay there and daydreamed of what it would be like to not have chronic pain. I think of all the things I could do or would be doing if I did not have fibromyalgia.

Most of my days are spent alone and I don't have a lot of distractions. Therefore, it gives me more time to indulge in these daydreams. It doesn't help anything or solve the pain, yet it seems a necessary part of the disease. Even though the outlook is bleak and the prognosis stays the same, there is always a part of me that appears hopeful. The days become weeks, the weeks become months, and eventually the months become years. Some days I can't believe I'm on my thirteenth year of fibromyalgia or chronic pain. It seems the more I know about the disease, the worse I get.

I try not to get too engrossed in these pity parties. Some days I'm just damn mad and I don't know what to do with it. I could scream, I could cry, I could throw a fit, but that doesn't help. If anything, all that would just cause me more pain. The problem is having a body that's failing, but having a mind that's healthy. I remember once reading where Farrah Fawcett said, "I feel like I'm a regular person just trapped in the shell of a body." That's how I feel. My mind goes places sometimes that my body can't. Sometimes in my dreams I'm well, with no pain and no worries.

Having a chronic pain condition and being unable to work are two really scary things. What if I had to provide for myself? What if I couldn't afford my medications? What if my friends and family were not so understanding? And of course, the really scary thought is what if I get worse? On nights I can't sleep, all of these questions run through my mind again and again. It just doesn't make any sense to have pain for no reason. Especially a pain that hurts so bad that sometimes I think I'd rather die than endure it. Just think about that for a minute. The pain that was so bad and so unbearable that you wish you were dead. It's not that I'm suicidal; I'm just desperate sometimes.

Everything I do in my everyday life is painful. To look at the list seems crazy to an average person. I truly think the only time I don't feel pain is when I'm asleep. On days when my pain is unbearable, like a ten plus, the only thing I can do is take something for sleep. It's like I have already crossed the line of no return. Even when I wake up, there are those few minutes before my brain wakes up that I don't have pain. However, once my brain wakes up so does the pain and there starts my day. Plus, I only get one cup of energy, so I better use it wisely. Next is going to be the list of things that cause me pain. I'm sure many people with fibromyalgia will agree with the list.

Everyday things that cause pain in people with fibromyalgia:

1. A pen that does not write smooth
2. Putting on makeup and fixing our hair
3. Shopping carts that don't roll easily
4. Sitting or standing more than five to ten minutes
5. Sitting through church or a movie
6. A door that's hard to open
7. Typing on the computer or texting on the phone
8. Using touch screens such as those at an ATM or photo shop.
9. Stress from holidays
10. Standing at the stove cooking or stirring a pot
11. Scooping ice cream
12. Lack of sleep or missing a nap
13. Twisting doorknobs or pulling the drawer out that doesn't open smoothly

14. Going to the hair salon and leaning back into the shampoo bowl, or sitting under the hairdryer
15. Trying to sleep with a noisy partner or having constant sleep disruptions
16. Pulling wet clothes out of the washer
17. Changing the fitted sheets on the bed
18. Making a left turn and having to turn your neck left-right-left
19. Pulling the trash bag out of the trash can with a fitted liner
20. Ironing or pressing clothes
21. Pushing buttons on a calculator or remote control
22. Hanging in a shower curtain or reaching over my head
23. Wrapping a gift
24. Opening any lid to a jar and trying to tear plastic open
25. Playing any card or board games, or reading books

I'm sure there're so many others that are not listed here, but I think people get the general idea that nearly everything we do causes pain.

Everyday Options that Can Make Your Life with FMS Easier

1. Go to stores where the doors open automatically.
2. Buy furniture that is lightweight and easy to move.
3. Wear shoes that are lightweight and slip on or off without laces or straps.
4. Riding in a truck or SUV than a car that may have bucket seats or very little leg room.
5. Take a nice easy walk either outside or in the mall, whichever keeps you comfortable.
6. Keep bottled water handy at all times so as not to get dehydrated.
7. Carry tennis balls in your purse to use as acupressure for long trips.
8. Be prepared to lie down anywhere if sitting becomes too painful.
9. Try a zero-gravity chair, the weightlessness can ease some of your painful pressure points.

10. When you are shopping for clothes, try to find ones with as few buttons and snaps as possible.
11. Try not to allow yourself to get too hot or too cold.
12. Consider putting a seat and a safety handle in your shower.
13. Avoid heavy coats, shoulder bags, and heavy blankets on your bed.
14. Listen to your own body and take care of "you." Make sure you always have medication with you, rest when you can, and don't be ashamed to say "I can't."

Chapter Eleven
Lost Wages and Broken Families

The subject of this chapter really concerns me, especially since there seem to be more people getting the diagnosis of FMS all the time. I don't have children so I can only imagine how difficult it would be to manage children under constant pain and fatigue. Having FMS has had a huge impact on my relationships and work. My first husband left me because he was tired of me being sick and tired. Six years ago, I was told I can no longer work. I was engaged at the time so my fiancé and I decided to go ahead and get married. We had already planned to get married, but had to move it up since I was going to have to rely on my husband's income and insurance. I was only forty years old and all of a sudden I can no longer work and support myself. Some people my age that have FMS do have children, they have to work, and they're practically killing themselves to keep their families going. Some of those people get little sympathy from their spouse and their employer.

What are we going to do with all these families that are struggling because one parent has fibromyalgia? How are we going to help the patients take care of their home and family? What about their ever-mounting medical bills and prescription expenses? How is the government going to handle all these otherwise healthy individuals suddenly unable to work? These are the questions we must be asking senators and congressmen. Will FMS patients get assistance or disability and how will they survive on disability alone? We are talking hundreds of thousands of people between the ages of twenty-five and fifty, mainly women, who suddenly cannot work. It worries me and it should worry the government of the United States. Maybe the medical community could help by recognizing that FMS is a painful and debilitating disease.

Then there are the broken families. Mothers unable to keep the household going and their children cared for. Maybe there is a young mother out there dealing with unrelenting pain and exhaustion and trying to care for a newborn. These and other situations like these have led to divorce, the patient and children moving in with relatives. I have even read stories where the FMS patient could not pay rent due to medical bills and had to be evicted. This is terrible. Some days, I want to scream to the world, "It's not our fault, we did not ask for this pain and hardship."

I know me personally, I would give anything to have my old life back, the life that was free of pain and fatigue and was able to work full-time. I know there are some out there who think not working is a luxury. Yeah, this is some luxury, having pain 24/7, fatigue so bad I can hardly get out of bed, not being able to enjoy shopping or going to the movies. I have had to discover a whole new "me," find new things to enjoy and coming to terms with my spiritual self. I have learned to stop the pity party and thank God for every day I have.

It didn't happen overnight. I had to learn to ask for help and I had to learn that I am worth it. We all are worthy of giving and receiving love no matter what illness we have. I used to get upset because people showed me very little sympathy for having FMS. Then I realized I don't need their sympathy and maybe they truly don't understand the disease fibromyalgia. I have the disease and some days I don't even understand it. FMS is very complicated and hard to explain. It's like any other disease. I don't have cancer so I have no idea what it feels like or how hard life with cancer is.

Chapter Twelve

I am not a medical doctor or expert on fibromyalgia, but based on things I've read, these things seem to have relevance.

1. Spinal stenosis or Chiari malformation
2. History of spinal injury or family history of spinal disease
3. Low growth hormone, or elevated substance P
4. History of a Major Depressive Episode
5. Trigger points or areas of tenderness in the muscles
6. Low pain threshold
7. Lack of restorative sleep
8. History of infection, examples like Lyme Disease and Infectious Mononucleosis
9. Raynaud's phenomenon
10. Chronic widespread pain for no apparent reason

I know there are other symptoms and possible disease correlation that could be added to this list. Every fibromyalgia patient is different, so how they got the disease and what their background is would pertain only to the individual. Also, as more research is done they will continue to find the importance of family history as well as the personal history of the patients themselves.

ACR Fibromyalgia Diagnostic Criteria

Fibromyalgia is a distinctive syndrome which can be diagnosed with critical precision. It may occur in the absence (primary fibromyalgia) or presence of other conditions such as rheumatoid arthritis or systemic lupus erythematosus (concomitant fibromyalgia). It is rarely secondary to another disease, in the sense that alleviation or the associated disease also cures the fibromyalgia. It may be confidently diagnosed in patients with widespread musculo-skeletal pain and multiple tender points.

The American College of Rheumatology 1990 Criteria for the Classification of Fibromyalgia

History of widespread pain has been present for at least three months.

Definition: Pain is considered widespread when all of the following are present:
- Pain in both sides of the body
- Pain above and below the waist. In addition, axial skeletal pain (cervical spine, anterior chest, thoracic spine or low back pain) must be present. Low back pain is considered lower segment pain.

Pain in 11 of 18 tender point sites on digital palpation

Definition: Pain, on digital palpation, must be present in at least 11 of the following 18 tender point sites:
- Occiput
  (2) - at the suboccipital muscle insertions
- Low cervical
  (2) - at the anterior aspects of the intertransverse spaces at C5-C7
- Trapezius
  (2) - at the midpoint of the upper border
- Supraspinature
  (2) - at origins, above the scapula spine near the medial border
- Second
  rib (2) - upper lateral to the second costochondral junction
- Lateral
  epicondyle (2) - 2 cm distal to the epicondyles
- Gluteal
  (2) - in upper outer quadrants of buttocks in anterior fold of muscle
- Greater
  trochanter (2) - posterior to the trochanteric prominence

- Knee
(2) - at the medial fat pad proximal to the joint line

Digital palpation should be performed with an approximate force of 4 kg. A tender point has to be painful at palpation, not just "tender."

Illustration of Tender Points

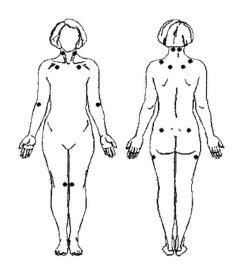

Fibromyalgia Syndrome Symptoms

Condition	% of FMS Symptoms
Muscular Pain	100
Fatigue	96
Insomnia	86
Joint Pains	72
Headaches	60
Restless Legs	56
Numbness and Tingling	52
Impaired Memory	46
Leg Cramps	42
Impaired Concentration	41
Nervousness	32
Depression (Major Depression)	20

File:Muscles anterior labeled.png

From Wikipedia, the free encyclopedia

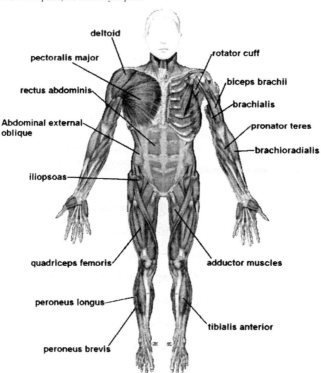

Size of this preview: 516 × 599 pixels
Full resolution (1,156 × 1,342 pixels, file size: 856 KB, MIME type: image/png)

 This is a file from the Wikimedia Commons. Information from its **description page there** is shown below.
Commons is a freely licensed media file repository. You can help.

Description

w:Collage of varius w:Gray's muscle pictures by Mikael Häggström (User:Mikael Häggström)

Fibromyalgia Syndrome

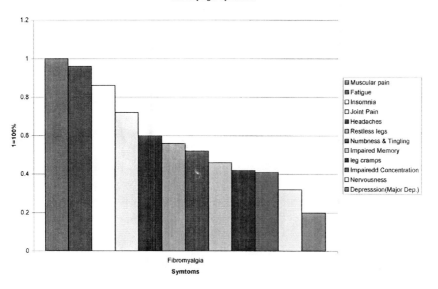